Self-Hypnosis

Learn Basic Techniques For

Personal Transformation

By

Meenakshi Narang

Table of Contents

INTRODUCTION

I immensely thank you for downloading this e-book. This informative e-book will act as a practical guide for you to understand the concept of hypnosis and self-hypnosis. Our mystical mind holds immense power to solve and resolve many of our complexes that tend to make our lives stressful. Hypnosis is all about putting our minds to deep sleep and taming it of its knots. Hypnosis, if effectively applied and practiced, can help in making our minds clearly focused. This e-book titled, 'Secrets for Hypnosis for

Beginners: Self Hypnosis Techniques that will transform you forever' includes some useful and effective techniques. Self-hypnosis has been explained in a simple and clear language so that a layman can understand them without hassles and apply the same. Those who are new to hypnosis and self-hypnosis will be able to learn about them in the simplest way. Just follow the step wise instructions and get rewarding results from them.

Happy Reading!

Chapter 1 –What is Hypnosis?

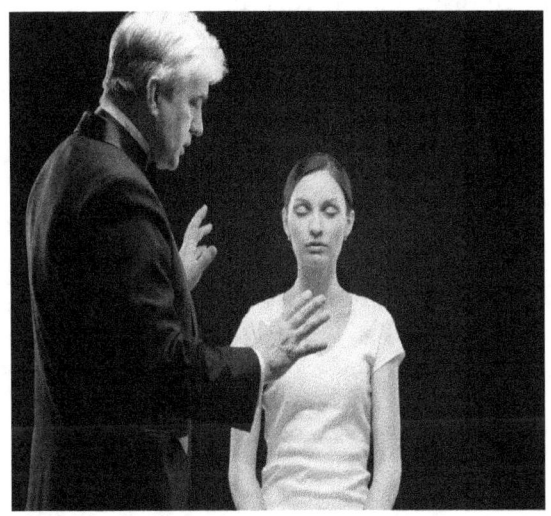

Hypnosis is a state of mind in its innate composure state and lays focus on selective things. Hypnosis allows conditioning of the mind that would allow healing for its many complexities. The practice of the hypnotizing mind is prevalent since time immemorial and has been practiced at various levels.

Our mind, in its subconscious state, is unable to explore its capabilities. By entering in a hypnotic state, one can delve deep in mind and attune it to the desired perceptions for bettering our thinking and behavior. Psychologists take help of clinical hypnosis for treating many patients of their mental and psychological disorders.

The characteristic of hypnosis are as follows:

- **Authorization**: A person cannot be hypnotized without his will and permission. Since, hypnosis is a direct interaction between the hypnotized person and hypnotists, there has to be a feeling of trust and loyalty between the two. This way the hypnosis can work out for whatever purpose it is being performed.

- **Imagination**: When a person achieves the state of hypnosis and, maintains it, the hypnotist can send ideas, advice and suggestion into the unconscious mind. Once the sent ideas are perceived by the hypnotized person he or she can accept those things that are basically a solution for his/her problems. After that, they will experience a lot of changes in life and thought process as well. For instance, an overweight person suffers mental as well as physical stress due to his low self-esteem his own body. But when the subconscious mind will accept the new perception and ideas, his thoughts and feelings about himself will automatically change. This is what hypnosis does; it changes the perspective of a person and initiates change in his life.

- **Concentration**: Concentration is all about focusing. When a person is hypnotized, he only listens and follows the voice of the hypnotist and nothing else. In other words, during this process the person is kept away from his experience of the world and is focused towards that particular stage of hypnosis.

- **Relaxation**: Mostly a person feels his eyes heavy and desires to relax. Being in the hypnotic state of mind makes a person feel good and stress-free.

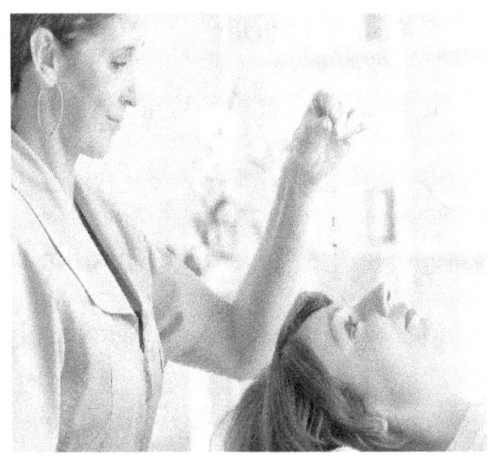

Connotations of Hypnosis

The term hypnosis has a number of meanings and definitions, depending on the experiments and research results made by many doctors and surgeons. The earliest definition related to hypnosis was introduced by James Braid, who assumed that hypnotism is nervous sleep and is completely different from normal sleep.

However, he further elaborated the same with his works and stated that the actual origin of hypnosis lies in mental concentration. When an individual is in the state of mental concentration, he becomes indifferent and unconscious about the rest of the world, others' thoughts and ideas. He gets inclined in a single idea or a train of thoughts and his intellect and mind doesn't think of any other thing beside the current thought that is being presented before him by hypnotist.

Chapter 2 - Self Hypnosis

'Self-hypnosis' quite resembles hypnosis but with only slight variation. The only difference between the two is, in hypnosis there is a person, often a hypnotist that hypnotizes the subject. And In self-hypnosis, we hypnotize ourselves with certain methods and techniques. There is no hypnotist who conducts the procedure thus acting as a medium or guide. Self Hypnosis involves all the process and procedure to be conducted by the subject himself or herself. It is highly used in modern hypnotherapy by many psychologist and doctors. It helps a person in relaxing himself entirely within a very short span of time thus reducing anxiety, sleeplessness, tiredness, and rebuilding confidence and self-esteem.

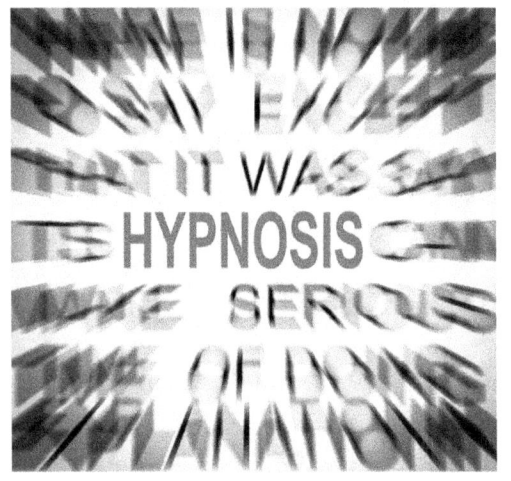

Self-Hypnosis vs. Hypnosis

It has been observed that mostly people prefer self-hypnosis rather than hypnosis. In many cases, if a person seeks help of a professional hypnotherapist, it is totally about what a self-hypnosis can do and what not. Self-hypnosis is undoubtedly a strong tool, but it has its limitations. A person, wanting to experience hypnosis, must be completely aware of all the aspects of both of these thus to decide the best choice. It is important to state here that hypnosis in any of its format must not be attempted if it is not understood or comprehended well. Since it involves the training and conditioning of mind, it becomes imperative to understand its nuances before implementing it.

In self-hypnosis, it is important to understand the complexity of the process involved. Some of the techniques are simple that can be started in around 3 to 4 breathes. State of deep relaxation is the main aim that a person does it for the same purpose. However, in hypnosis, it is more focused, more suggestible and more disassociated from the rest of the world.

But eventually, both self hypnosis and hypnosis can make a person happy and stress-free. Hypnosis if used by hypnotherapist in order to detach people from problem causing emotions and try to focus them to find more wider and possibilities to remain happy and calm. Whereas, in self-hypnosis, which resembles meditation, people recall and rename their feelings but do not attach themselves with them, as a result of which they experience many benefits.

Hypnosis is used as a therapy that generally focuses a person to relax even if he is surrounded by memories and prepares to feel and think positive desiring to act differently from the past, in the upcoming future. So as the self hypnosis do.

Chapter 3 - Self Hypnosis Techniques For Beginners

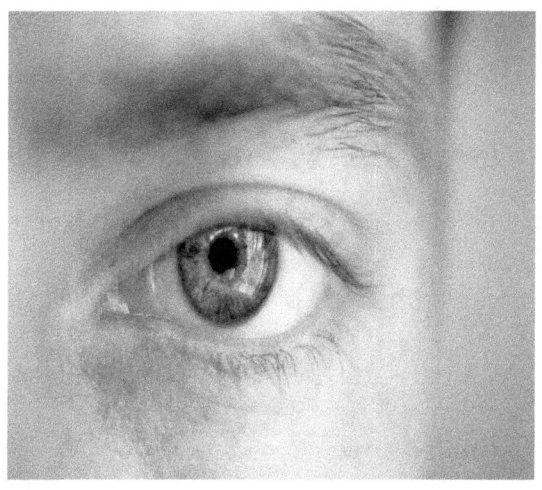

There are many sessions involve in teaching self hypnosis to beginners. However, initially it teaches beginners to relax and to stay calm. Without learning the relaxation, one cannot move further to achieve self hypnosis goals. Here are some steps for learning relaxation -

• At the initial stage, a person should remember and recall a trigger word like some familiar ones as 'sunshine' or 'beach'. One can also try to remember a place where once he visited and felt very relaxed and calmed down.

• Next step is to take deep breathe from the stomach as we do during the time of falling asleep. However, bedtime is the best time to practice self hypnosis techniques.

- Once you learn to breathe deep, think of yourself in relaxing mode so that you can go ahead with self hypnosis

How self-hypnosis is helpful?

Self-hypnosis is very useful in numerous problems. It bears a power to rectify all sorts of problem. It is a medium for stress relief and self-improvement. It is slightly different from mediation as mediation tends to become passive and generalized while self hypnosis is focused on a particular goal. In mediation a person is just concentrated on breathing or some chanting but in self hypnosis person focuses on suggestions and imaginations to be visualized for self-improvement. On the whole, if positive thoughts and visualization are combined it becomes self hypnosis. It helps people in reducing their pain, anxiety, and depressions. Besides, it sorts out problems related to physical body and help in quitting bad habits like smoking and drinking. Some of the uses of self hypnosis are mentioned below:

Instant stress relief: It helps to have instant stress relief from everyday life for getting relief from all sorts of tensions. The mind and the body experience levels of freedom from many sorts of complexes that often mar our peace of mind. A person is required to take deep breath and along with that the heart also slows down. It speeds up again when person inhales. This regular and irregular heart beat indicates that there is a healthy interaction between the heart and mind. It works like- inhale and heart beat is faster; exhale and heart beat becomes slower. This helps a lot in reduction of stress.

Self-improvement: This is further divided into three sub parts as: achievement, concentration and peak performance; that enable to get better results. The three of them are given in brief as below:

a) **Achievement:** In self hypnosis, it firstly takes you to motivational level to do anything that lies within your comfort zone, and even outside that. Source for motivation can be fear or stress, or it can be excitement or fun of working with one's hobby. The positive motivation helps to improve our working ability and building up

24

our self-confidence to perform any kind of task with greater efficiency. It actually energizes us.

b) **<u>Concentration:</u>** It is the most important thing that everyone needs to furbish for better performance. A person performs his best when he is completely concentrated on a task and not distracted with any of the wavering thoughts and useless ideas. Mostly, whatever we do, we don't like and fail to concentrate and motivate. Generating motivation with self hypnosis becomes a little bit tough, but it can be overcome with the subconscious mind involved in self hypnosis method.

c) **Peak performance:** This is what is resulted after achievement and concentration. A person becomes perfect to attain unmatchable performance putting his best in the same with lots of enthusiasm and excitement. He now becomes the best performer no matter what task he has to do., He performs everything with great passion, concentrated over his goals and without being distracted.

Confidence and self-esteem: Self-esteem is what a person thinks and feels about him. In other words person with a low self-esteem is said to have inferiority complex whereas the one with high self-esteem bears a superiority complex. But extreme cases are dangerous for an individual. However, low self-esteem indicates that a person has low confidence. He is more insecure about him and his capabilities. But with self hypnosis all this can be sorted out. It teaches an individual to believe in himself, and he enlists all the good qualities of him that he can offer to

27

society and world. Being grateful and being good to you can increase the self-esteem and self-confidence. Eventually, a person should love and respect him before anyone in this world. This would render many positive results and better state of mind.

Weight loss: Self hypnosis is the best mental workout for weight loss. In order to do dieting and exercises, there is need of lot of motivation and positive thinking in order to keep up the spirit. This can be achieved with self hypnosis that motivates to eat right and helps to overcome negativity regarding an individuals' body image. Self-hypnosis also acts a motivator and confidence booster to lose weight. There are several guidelines that a person must follow with great enthusiasm and passion. There should be no starving, intake of proper and balanced diet, exercising, etc Setting of such achievable goals at initial stage, and most importantly usage of self hypnosis techniques has been rendering better and long lasting effects.

Maintaining healthy relationships: Everyone faces challenges and certain problems in relationships at some stage of life. Therefore, self hypnosis is extremely helpful in concentrating positive beliefs and healthy attitude towards a relationship. It develops a person's mind and perception in such a manner that he starts to understand likes and dislikes of partner and accepts them as they are. They begin to understand that no matter how much a person loves and cares for another, he can't get to know needs and wants of partner until he will not speak up. Thus, one learns to open up and talk about his feelings freely to his partner.

Release of addiction (smoking, drinking, and drug addiction): Numerous people use self hypnosis to quit the habit of smoking, drinking, and drug addiction. However, all this is a game of will power and correct use of self hypnosis. A person himself should want to leave such habits and not on the request of his partner or doctor. Only then, the process of hypnosis will work effectively. It provides instant relief from any sort of addiction.

Release of depression: Self hypnosis helps a lot in releasing depression. If a person always perceives and thinks the negative aspect of everything and situations, he is in serious depression, and there needs are some effective way to steer him out from depression. Self-hypnosis helps in teaching a person to look at the always positive side of a thing.

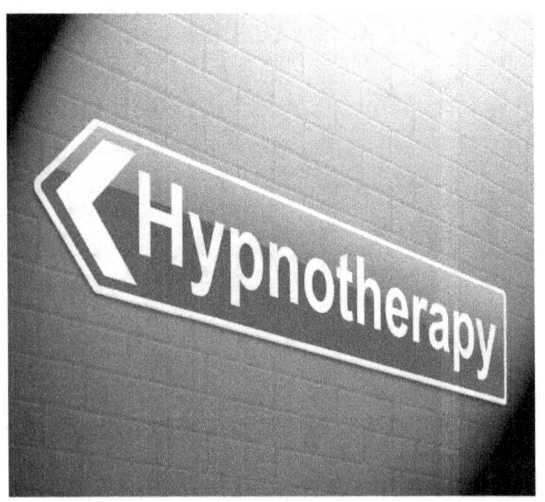

Techniques of Self Hypnosis

Self-hypnosis is a psychological state of mind that naturally happens and allows a person to achieve strengthened and focused concentration level. Apart from that it also help in changing belief system from negative to positive, gets rid of bad habits and addictions, and transforms the whole personality of a person. It also relaxes and de-stresses an individual from everyday life's worries and tensions, and keep up the motivation level high. Here are some techniques for performing self hypnosis correctly:

33

Step 1: Preparation for hypnosis:

- It is quite tough to enter in a deep and relaxed state of mind, but there needs to a strong will power that help one to avoid any distraction. One should be in very comfortable and easy clothing and ensure that the temperature of the place where he/she is going to perform self hypnosis is appropriate.

- A person must find a quiet and noise free room and sit in a comfortable chair, couch or even a bed. He can lie down as it is obvious that he will fall asleep after the self hypnosis. But one should keep in mind, whatever be the posture of the subject, one doesn't have to cross legs or any part of the body as that may become an obstacle in self hypnosis.

• The amount of time a person wants to dedicate to self hypnosis should be nominal as initially one cannot sit for a long time in the hypnotized state. Another important concern is to ensure complete seclusion. There should be no disturbance till the process of self hypnosis is going on. Gradually, you can increase the time of process as you become habitual and practiced self-hypnotist

• There should be certain goals and aims in the mind of the person who wants to do self hypnosis. The goal can be to relax the mind, for improving self-esteem and boost self-confidence, or it can be for achieving specific goals like quitting smoking and weight loss, etc. It can also result into some revolutionary changes into life. All depends on the person who is initiating self hypnosis. For example, if he wants to quit a smoking habit he must think about the lines "I do not want to smoke", "cigarettes are injurious to health and they cause cancer". Similarly, if someone wants to lose his or her weight the lines like 'I eat healthily, and I am losing my weight" should be recited.

Step 2: Entering into hypnosis:

- At the time of entering hypnosis, it might be difficult to think or focus, and a person will observe that thoughts are continuously getting interrupted. However, do not force thoughts. Rather, allow them to flow freely. Don't let yourself indulge in them. If you like to focus on a point in a wall or somewhere else, do it with concentrating on eyelids. Keep on telling you that the eyelids are getting heavier, and they cannot remain open anymore.

• Afterward, feel that all parts of the body are becoming lighter, and all the tensions and worries are melting. Concentrate on toes, relax them and continue same with all parts of the body like calves, thighs, hips, stomach, till whole body starts feeling relaxed and lighter. If techniques like the use of warm water can soothe and comfort feet and ankles, use them effectively.

• While exhaling, monitor and observe the outflow of tension and negativity from your body. At the time of inhalation, feel the inflow of energy and positivity in your body. Imagine different kinds of things like a half-cut lemon and the taste of its juice. Get detailed visualization and think about all the five senses.

• Now that you are extremely relaxed and calmed down, feel and appreciate the situation. Imagine yourself on ten stairs where the water starts from the 5th stair, and as you move downward water begins to touch your feet, making you feel refreshing and very cool. Then start to feel that water is getting higher towards your body. At this stage, the heart will start beating faster. However, experience the sound, sight and feel of clean, fresh and pure water.

• On reaching the bottom of the water, feel a sensation of floating. If you are unable to perceive the feeling try again by concentrating and visualizing. Afterward, start describing your feeling and experiences silently only to yourself.

• You can repeat all the statements as many times as you like and feel refreshed. Feel free and wandering in the water. Imagine yourself to be empty boxes placed inside the water and finding treasure. It would appear as if you are finding money, self-confidence, and self-esteem and discarding all the tensions. Continue to imagine and find where the water is cold, hot or full of life.

• Moreover, now prepare yourself to exit the state of hypnotism. With each

41

step you move upward, feel like water is going lower, and you have again reached the fifth stair. When you have stopped visualizing all those things, give yourself a minute or two to open eyes. Imagine that the light is pouring through the doorway, and this would make your eyes open naturally. Take some time while getting up and tell yourself again and again 'wide awake'.

Step 3: Enhance and Expand your Experience

- If you don't believe in self hypnosis, no technique will ever work out in real life. A person should have to believe in him and his actions only then this technique will help out. In fact, one should write down all the experience that he had while performing self hypnosis. If it wasn't very effective at the initial stage, give yourself some time and practice. Try this after few days and recall the experiences you might get surprised.

• Believe in yourself and open your entire mind that will promote working out of this method in a proper manner. Any negative thought will hinder the path of progress of self-hypnotism.

• If a person needs to know if he is in a trance or not there are some exercises to check the same. Twine fingers together and tell yourself that that they are stuck together. Now try to take them apart. If this cannot be done, it proves that you are in trance.

• Assume that your one arm is getting heavier, and you don't need to bear it's weight. The brain will automatically do this for you. Try to lift it up. If you can't, it proves yet again.

- Be confident and think positively about whatever you are dedicated to. Visualize yourself in the situation and try to find out that how are you reacting in that situation. For losing the weight imagine yourself in perfectly skinny and tight jeans, the model before the mirror, and smile at your beautiful and spectacular body.

- Some people like to have music as a trigger for self hypnosis. Imagine yourself wandering about the whole world smiling, and making eye contact with people. This can help you become extrovert and get rid of shy nature.

- Use self hypnosis to better yourself and improve your self-esteem. Determine a goal you would to like to achieve and concentrate over that during the relaxed state of mind. Envisage the person you want to be and try to become that kind of person. Self-hypnosis is very helpful for deep meditation and can be used for bigger and better purposes. It is right to choose self hypnosis to get rid of bad habits, change belief system, perceptions and to focus on goals of life more considerably.

- Another self hypnosis technique is to get back to some past mood or state of mind when the level of your confidence was upbeat and lofty. The self hypnosis will help in attaining the same state of mind. Just think and visualize about those bygone days and experience same moods. Create a mental picture where you are living in the past. Feel same and similar emotions so that the past can be relived. Visualize and experience them with such conviction that as if you have brought back your past.

- If your low phase is going on, tune up things several notches higher, try the technique of turning up the things higher. Once the right kind of mood has been created, imagine that you are turning up the intensity of a dial. Imagine it to be the dial of your motivation level and confidence. As you would move the dial up, feel as if the new zeal of motivation is getting infused in you. Whenever you find yourself to be slipping back into oblivion, tune up the dial again.

Chapter 4: More Practical Techniques

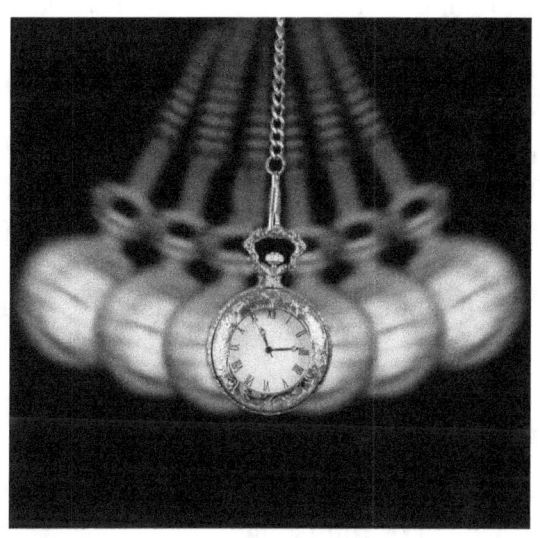

Relaxation Technique

Hypnotic state cannot be reached until mind and body are relaxed. A worried mind and a terse body cannot attain a hypnotic state. Thus relaxation technique is very important to make your mind tranquil and restful. Follow the listed to practice relaxation technique that would aid in self hypnosis -

- Locate an appropriate object that would help you in focusing your vision and mental stance. The object should be slightly elevated from you're the height of your sight.

- Soothe your mind and keep it cleared of any thoughts. Focus on the selected object. The mind will possibly be distracted initially, and jump like monkey, but gradually it would get settled with little practice and patience.

• Lay your attention on your eyes and feel your eyelids. Imagine that they are getting heavier. Breathe slowly and focus while you inhale and exhale.

• As you intensify your breathing, relax even further. Gradually slow down your breathing and watch your every breath.

• If the object is a pendulum, the hypnotic state will be achieved faster. See the object from your mind's eye and allow the perception to go deeper into your psyche.

- Start counting from 1 to 10 in mind and repeat the phrase "I am relaxing" with every count. Carry the belief that moment you will reach the count of 10, your mind is going to be in the hypnotic state.

- Just as you reach the hypnotic state of mind, concentrate on the personal goal or the statement that you have thought. Percept it in your mind and repeat it again and again. All the while, stay relaxed and focused.

- Chant the positivity as you count further. After reaching the count of 10, start back slowly. Follow the reversal process and again speak a positive message that would help you become better. You will wake up energetically with a revived mind.

Instant Age Regression Technique

Feeling the age regression can be done via instant self-hypnotic technique. It is all about getting rid of our mental blockades and complexities that are deep rooted into our past. Follow the listed points that would build up the base for instant technique -

- Close your eyes and think about your past life. In your mind, follow the timeline of your past life. Go in descending order, that is, imagine in your mind the incidents that happened just day before. Gradually, move towards thinking about last week, last month, and last year, and so on.

- This will help you in making your mind attuned to the sense of time. Now make a switchover and think about your future in the same format.

Close your eyes and think of all those things that you are likely to do tomorrow onwards, and then next week, next month and so on.

- Once the timeline gets established, use it to condition your mind in an advantageous way. Just float along your timeline and enjoy it along. Enjoy your happy past or float in future to do all things that you are aspiring for.

- Imagine a wide and a spacious road where you would be able to fit all that your want. Imagine you are standing on the timeline with a flagpole posted at your present moment. This image will help you stay rooted.

• Recall back the smells, sights and experiences that would bring in the happy memories to your mind. Gradually, your senses would join your mind in recalling back all the perception.

• This practice will help in overcoming some hard challenges pertaining to your work, personal situation, an event, some competition, an exam, or perhaps an interview.

• Now, close your eyes and imagine yourself standing on the timeline.

Imagine the future track and percept that you have overcome the challenge with positivity floating in the future. Experience the great satisfaction that comes after overcoming the satisfaction.

- Transport yourself to the achieving moment and witness your happiness and contentment.

- Now, float yourself backward and experience the results of this wonderful technique.

Self-Conversational Technique

- The conversational technique for self hypnosis follows simple and effective steps that render many desired benefits.

- It is important to get prepared for conversational technique by getting relaxed. Take deep breaths and allow your mind to get stable and focused.

- The conversational technique need not be done in an exhibiting manner. It can be done while sitting or just standing. This way the subject will not become a center of attraction.

- Loosen up your shoulders and nape of the neck. Feel the relaxation traveling down your spine and reaching towards your torso, buttocks, legs and your toes.

- Imagine your body to melt. Relax your stance and soften your demeanor. The idea is to relax, the primary requisite of self hypnosis.

- The objective behind conversational technique can be to sell some point or justification to persuade your mind and psyche.

- Get into the conversation with your own self and talk to yourself softly. Another option could be to listen to someone else and use his or her tone to hypnotize yours.

- Let others' words soothe your mind and dwell you mind over those things that are of interest to you.

- The conversational technique works best in those conditions where the boring conversation is going on where there is an exchange of repeated dialogs in a droning way.

Chapter 5 - Putting Yourself Into A Trance

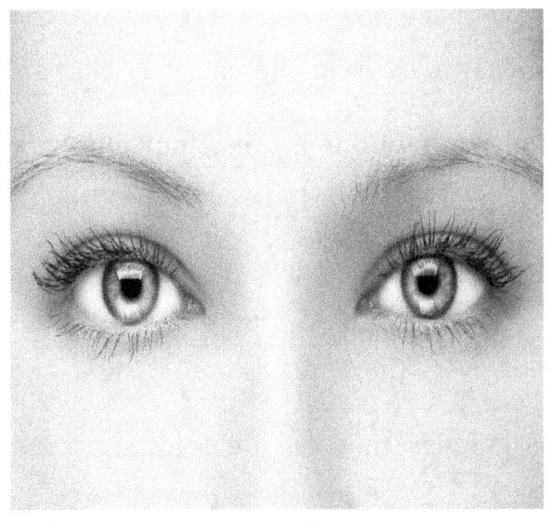

Trance refers to the hypnotic state of mind. There isn't anything unnatural about trance as it is a tranquil space where mind relaxes and allows delving deep into it perceptions. In self hypnosis, it is important to put yourself in the trance in a proper way. It is not about going asleep; rather the subject may appear to be asleep but in a very alert and agile state of mind. Every individual may take different time to get in a trance.

However, there are some basic trance techniques that can be selected as per suitability. To begin with select a quiet place that is away from the hum drum. Arrange for a comfortable chair and sit on it in a relaxed manner. Start deep breathing and relax your mind and body.

Eye Fixation

Keep your eyes wide open and create focus on any object or point that is positioned above the line of your sight. Clear your mind of all distractions and stare that object. Breathe slowly and guide your mind to relax. Imagine your eyes getting heavier, and drowsy. Soon your mind will be alert but eyes may get closed, taking you in deep trance.

Utilizing Anxiety & Distractions

If it is tough to soothe your mind, allow your anxiety to take you into the trance state. Close your eyes and think about those times when your life was simpler and calmer. Allow your mind to travel backward and visualize those memory flashes. Soon your mind will relax and awaken your sub-consciousness.

Visualizing

Visualization is a significant method to get transported into the trance. Close your eyes and relax yourself. It could be anything like - taking a stroll on the beach, swimming in a river, or walking deep down into a forest. Think freely and loosen your mind and body to enter trance.

Imagery

Certain imageries are very effective in triggering trance state. Imagine you are standing on the upper side of a staircase and overlooking a heavenly site that is at the bottom. Now imagine you are climbing each stair one by one reaching to that wonderful site. As you would imagine descending, your mind will start loosening its knots and get in a hypnotic trance.

Getting into a trance cannot be accomplished in a debut session. It may take some time and effort to know what would work. For some, a single technique may work or a combination as per the suitability.

Getting out of trance

Do not panic over how to get out of trance. You must be equally relaxed and calm to come out of hypnosis. Do not assume that you would be fast asleep and oblivious to your surroundings. Your mind will keep very alert, and you would be able to fathom what is going inside your mind. To come out of trance, start counting backward and say something suitable to yourself like –

"After I finish back counting, my eyes will open to make me fresh and awake."

Dos and Don'ts

➤ Don't pick a varying time during day or night for self hypnosis. Stick to one particular time for better mental conditioning.

➤ Don't lie down else you may fall asleep

➤ Don't get worried if you are unable to get into a trance state. Hypnosis indeed demands practice and patience.

➤ Do maintain continuity and consistency in using self-hypnotic tapes

➤ Don't panic if you start forgetting what you heard even a minute back. This indicates that your mind is responding to hypnosis by ignoring the input.

➤ Do take help of slow and soothing music to focus or to ward off external distractions

➤ Don't force your mind to get into trance. The harder you would try, the mind would refuse to relax.

- Don't use domineering or overpowering hypnotic suggestions lest your mind would deflect those.

- Do keep your motivational level high and work over single issue

- Do establish a connection between your mind and body

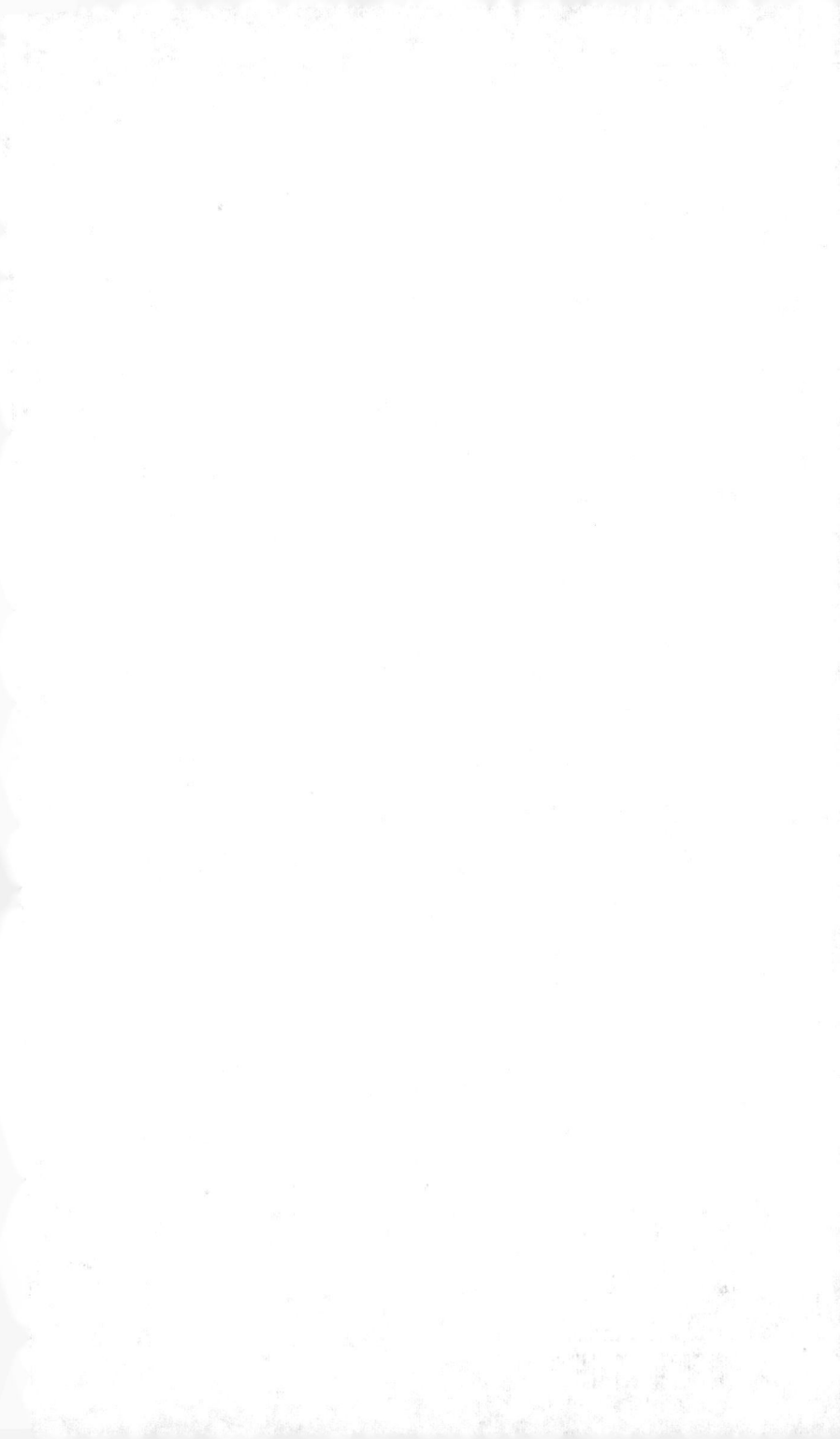